T0228657

Flourish

A Journey of Healing and Growth

HarperCollins*Publishers*
1 London Bridge Street
London SE1 9GF

www.harpercollins.co.uk

HarperCollins*Publishers*
Macken House, 39/40 Mayor Street Upper
Dublin 1, D01 C9W8, Ireland

First published by HarperCollins*Publishers* 2024

1 3 5 7 9 10 8 6 4 2

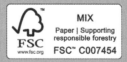

MIX
Paper | Supporting
responsible forestry
FSC™ C007454

This book is produced from independently certified FSC™ paper to
ensure responsible forest management.

For more information visit: www.harpercollins.co.uk/green

Flourish

A Journey of Healing and Growth

Steph Edwards

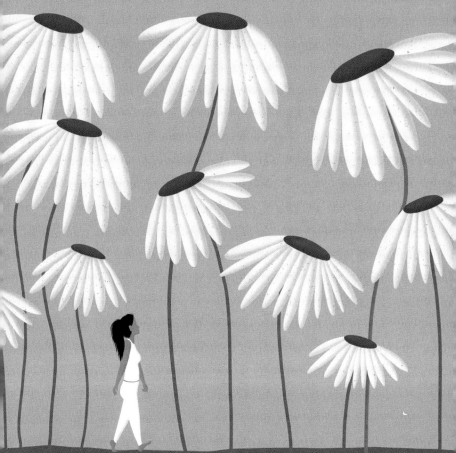

This book is dedicated to the most inspirational woman in my life, the person who not only gave me my creativity but also nurtured and encouraged it from the get-go. She is my biggest cheerleader, my best friend and the greatest teacher I ever had.

This one's for you, Mum.

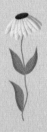

Contents

About me

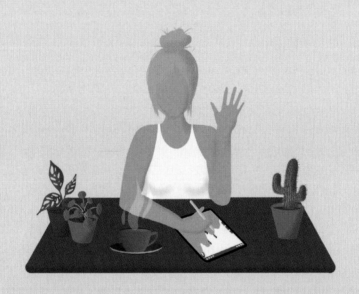

If you're reading this, whether it be in the bookstore, in your comfy reading chair at home, you're taking a cheeky peek at your friend's book, or it's been left on a park bench by mistake (I hope not!), then I'd like to say a massive thank you for being here!

So, who is the person behind the artwork? That'd be me, the waving blonde opposite. Hi, I'm Steph! An illustrator and all-round creative storyteller from a small village in Lancashire, England. I'm a tea-drinking chatterbox who uprooted her life in 2019 and moved to the Netherlands for love. I also created this book while pregnant with my first child, and I'm so excited to step into the next chapter of my life with my partner, Guido.

This journey all began back in 2021, when I tried out illustration as a way of creating a safe and supportive online space during COVID-19. But oh, it became so much more than just that. As a feminist, I wanted to create a space for women, I wanted to empower women, support women, lift them up and motivate them. I wanted my Instagram account to become a community for all women, everywhere.

My messages resonated with so many that I was lucky enough to turn my passion into a business: To You From Steph. You can find me over on Instagram (@toyoufromsteph) where I regularly create new artwork, share my life and hang out with the community I've built, come say hi! Or you can find my web shop online at toyoufromsteph.com where I sell my art on a variety of products, and where you can also read the whole story of how all of this began!

Growth

Buckle up, because we're diving headfirst into the grand adventure of becoming the best versions of ourselves. I mean, think about it - life is this crazy rollercoaster, and while we can't control all the twists and turns, we sure as heck can choose how we show up for the ride. So, welcome to the journey where you're both the passenger and the driver, the explorer and the mapmaker.

I always try to remind myself that self-growth isn't some mystical destination you stumble upon while wandering lost in the woods. It's more like a series of pit stops along the highway of life. It's those moments when you pause, look in the rearview mirror and go, 'Wow, I've come a long way'. It's the little things you do each day that accumulate into something big and beautiful.

Now, working on yourself is a wonderful accomplishment but it's not always sunshine and rainbows. Working on myself has been like holding a mirror up and really embracing every inch of who I am. The good, the bad and the ugly. It's about being one hundred per cent honest with myself about what makes me, me. Even if I don't like some of it. It's about finding those ugly inches and working out why they exist and how I can alter them for the better. Growth has become about communication, accountability, honesty and reflection.

Frankly, change can be downright uncomfortable. It's like wearing a new pair of shoes that pinch at first but eventually become your most comfortable kicks. Self-growth means stepping out of your comfort zone and daring to embrace the unfamiliar. Growth can mean that you realise unhealthy patterns, toxic people and places you no longer fit into. It's all part of your journey, and sometimes the excess luggage needs to be left behind.

Here's the beauty of it all: you're a work in progress, and that's something to be proud of. Self-growth isn't about perfection; it's about embracing the wild, wonderful ride along the way.

IT'S TIME TO SHED
WHAT HOLDS US BACK

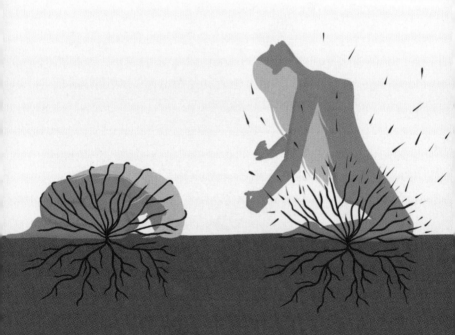

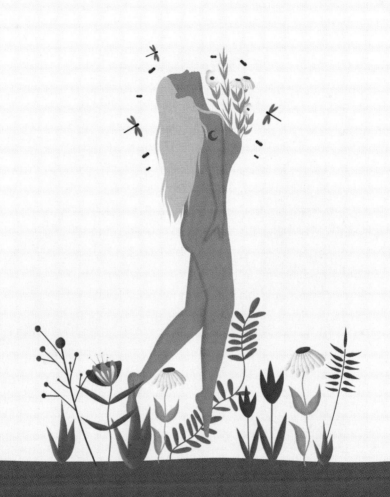

& FLOURISH

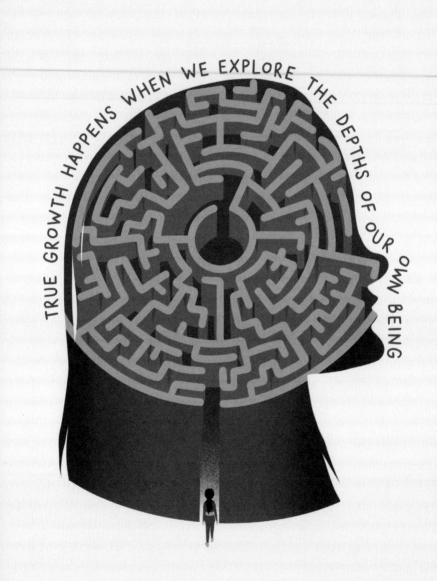

TRUE GROWTH HAPPENS WHEN WE EXPLORE THE DEPTHS OF OUR OWN BEING

GROWTH IS NOT LINEAR

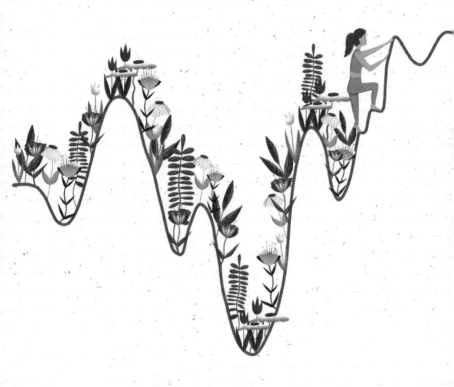

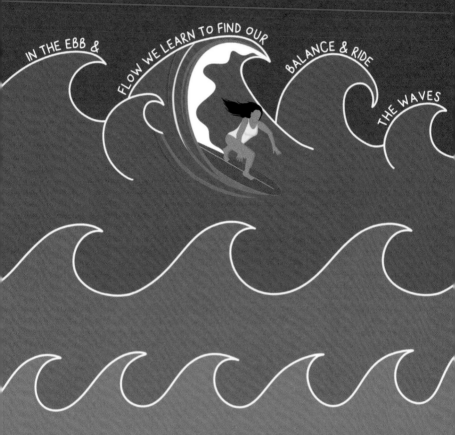

IN THE EBB & FLOW WE LEARN TO FIND OUR BALANCE & RIDE THE WAVES

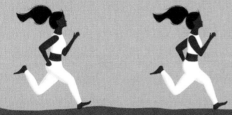

When you change,
don't announce it ...

JUST BLOOM

ALLOW YOURSELF TO GROW
AT YOUR OWN PACE

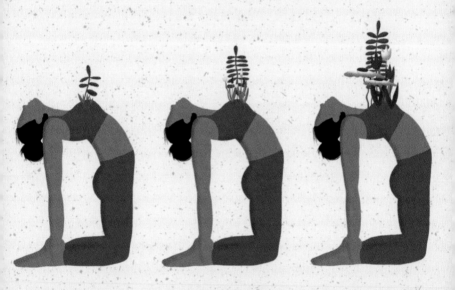

EVERY NOW AND THEN, IN THE DEPTHS OF OUR PAST

WE CAN FIND PEARLS OF WISDOM

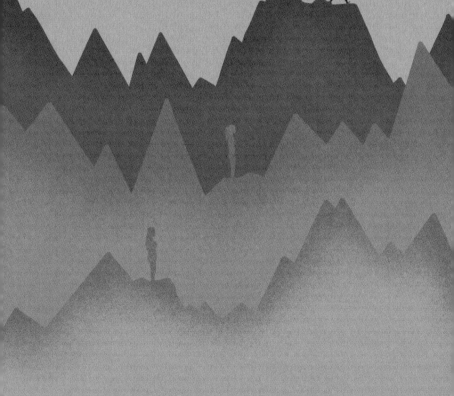

NOT EVERYONE WE MEET CAN WALK
THE WHOLE PATH WITH US & THAT'S OKAY

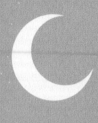

THERE IS COURAGE IN BEING AFRAID

BUT

PUSHING

FORWARD

ANYWAY

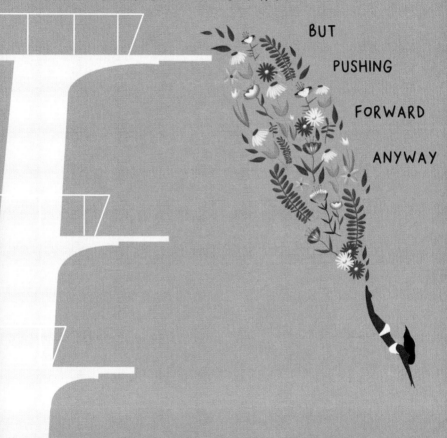

Amidst the darkness, it is easy to believe

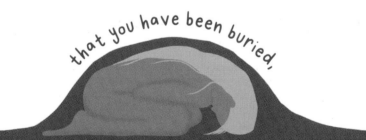

that you have been buried,

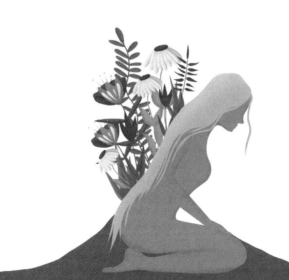

when really you've been planted

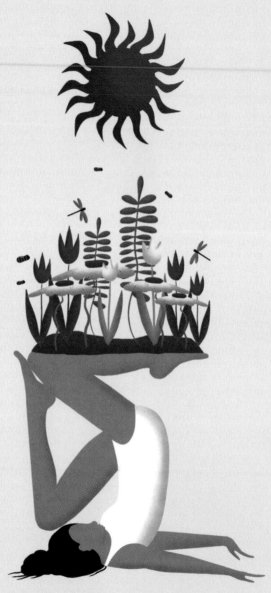

GROW WITH THE FLOW

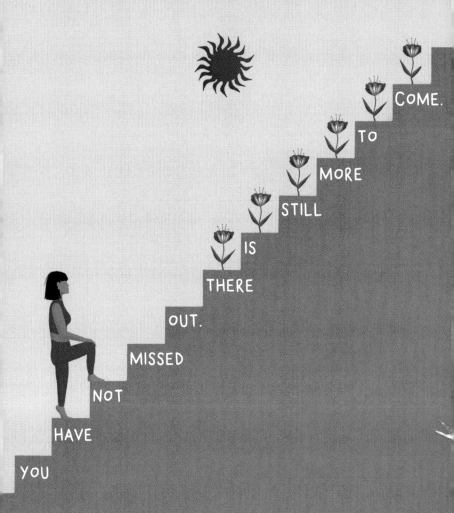

YOU
HAVE
NOT
MISSED
OUT.
THERE
IS
STILL
MORE
TO
COME.

The waves didn't get
smaller...

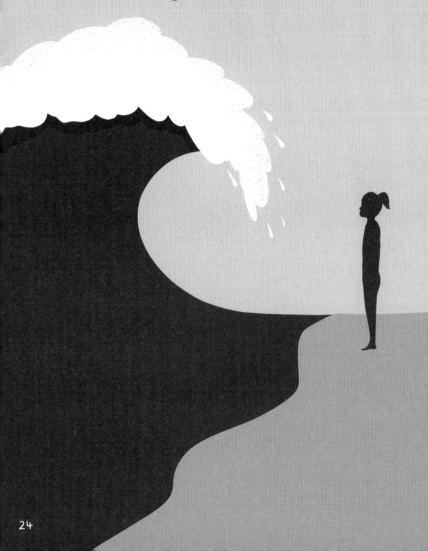

... I just grew and saw
them for what they were

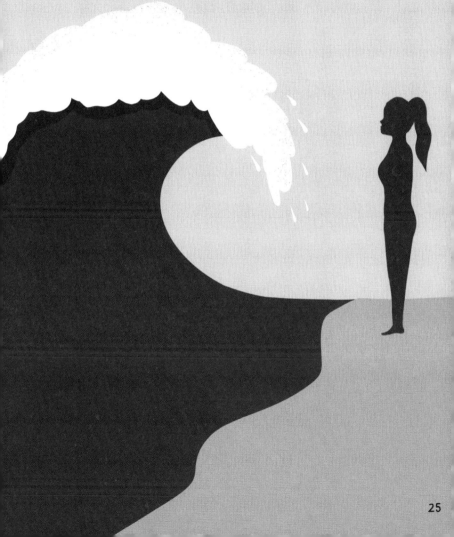

Healing

We've all stumbled, fallen or downright face-planted into moments that left us shattered; whether from heartbreak, loss or the battles we fight within ourselves. But here's the kicker: healing isn't about erasing those scars or pretending they never existed. Nope, it's about stitching ourselves back together with threads of resilience and self-compassion.

Picture this: you're a mosaic, made up of the beautiful shards of your experiences. Some gleam with brilliance, catching the light just right. Others, well, they bear the marks of storms weathered and lessons learned. Healing is about arranging those pieces into a kaleidoscope of strength - a patchwork that tells a story not just of pain, but of your incredible capacity to mend.

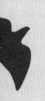

Let's get real here. Healing isn't skipping through a daisy covered field. It's more like stumbling through a dense forest, thorns and all. It's messy, it's non-linear, and at times, it feels like you're retracing the same painful steps over and over. But, oh, the magic lies in those moments when you pause, catch your breath and realise that the air smells a bit fresher, the sunlight filters through the leaves a bit softer.

We live in a world that's all about speed - fast internet, quick meals, instant messaging. But healing? Healing scoffs at the rush. It demands patience and the willingness to sit with discomfort. It's in those quiet moments of reflection, when you let yourself feel the depths of your emotions, that true healing begins to work its subtle wonders.

And guess what? You're not alone in this journey. Just as we all experience struggles, every soul has known the touch of pain and the need for healing. So, as we dive into this exploration of healing, let's do it with kindness, understanding and a whole lot of self-love. Because healing isn't about erasing the past - it's about crafting a future where you're stronger, wiser and more beautifully flawed than ever before.

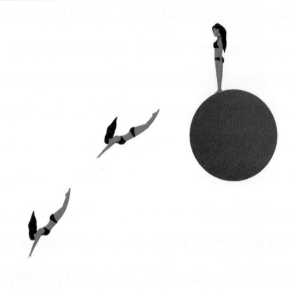

WHEN YOU'RE WILLING TO FEEL IT,

YOU CAN HEAL IT

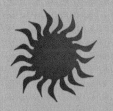

SOME STORMS

COME TO CLEAR YOUR

PATH AND GUIDE YOU

TO BRIGHTER DAYS

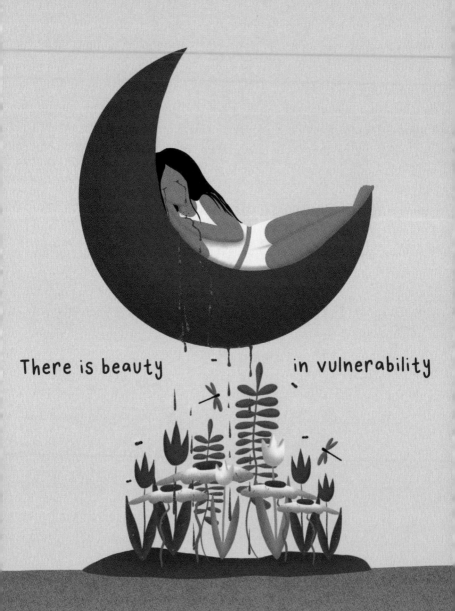

There is beauty — in vulnerability

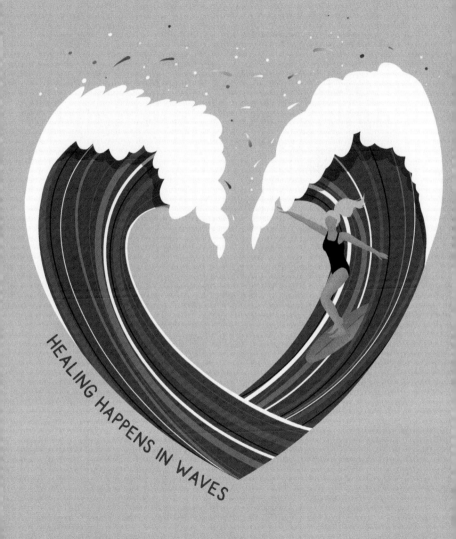

HEALING HAPPENS IN WAVES

If you're not speaking it, you're storing it, and that can feel heavy. Let it out

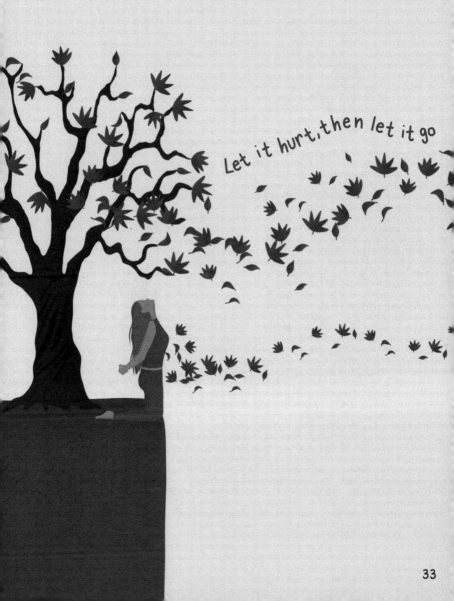

Let it hurt, then let it go

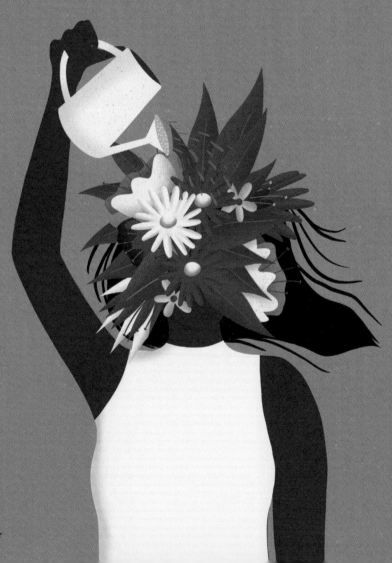

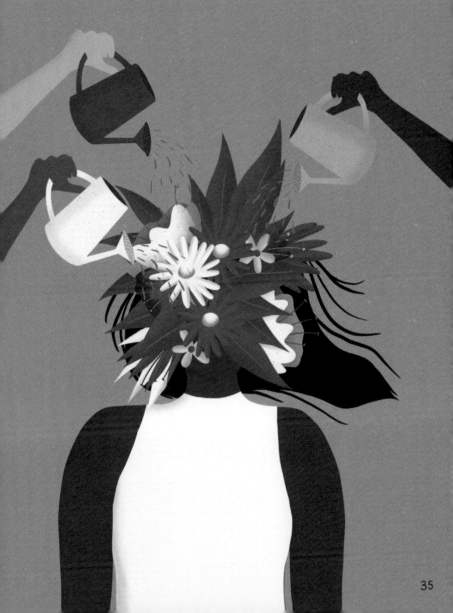

& OTHERS ARE FOR ACCEPTING HELP IN THE PROCESS

35

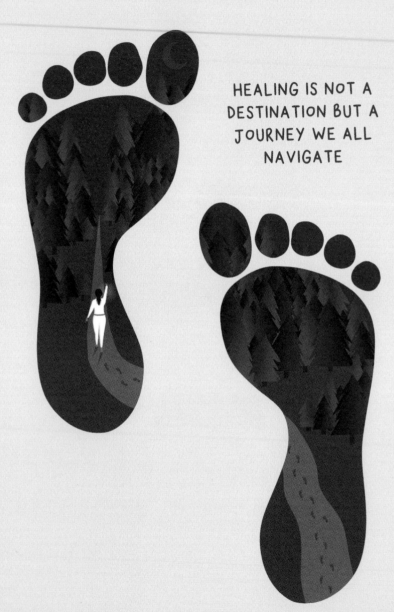

HEALING IS NOT A
DESTINATION BUT A
JOURNEY WE ALL
NAVIGATE

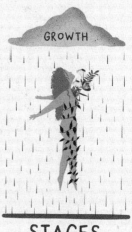

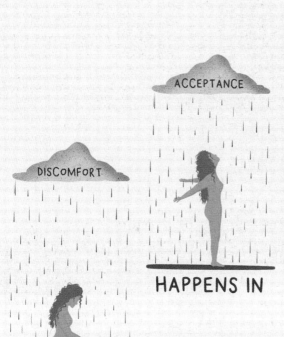

DISCOMFORT

ACCEPTANCE

GROWTH

HEALING

HAPPENS IN

STAGES

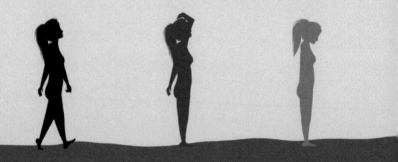

The moon reminds me that no matter

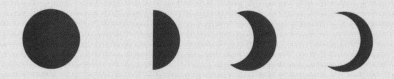

what phase I am going through ...

... I AM ALWAYS WHOLE

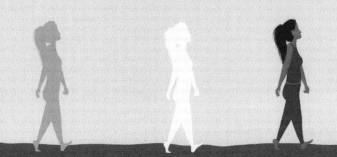

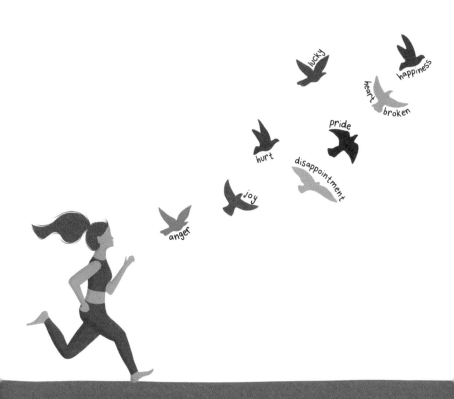

GIVE YOURSELF PERMISSION TO <u>FEEL HOW YOU FEEL</u>

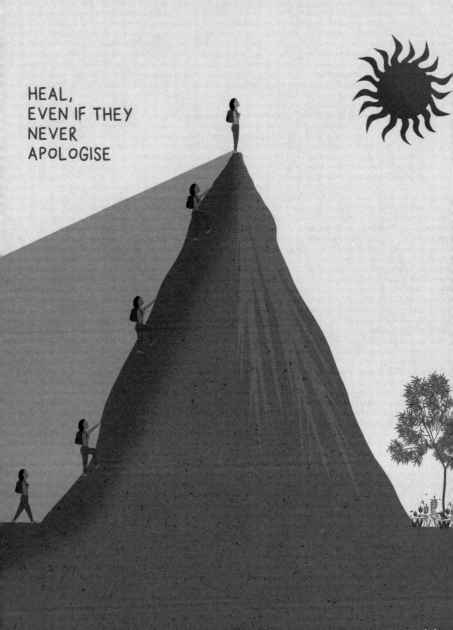

HEAL,
EVEN IF THEY
NEVER
APOLOGISE

41

Talking helps

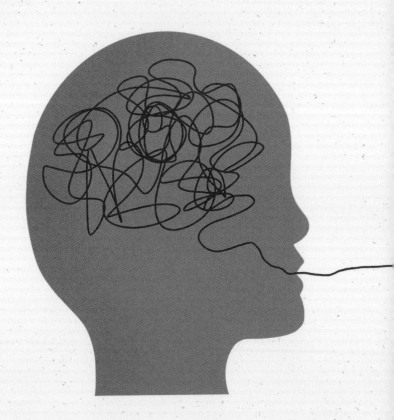

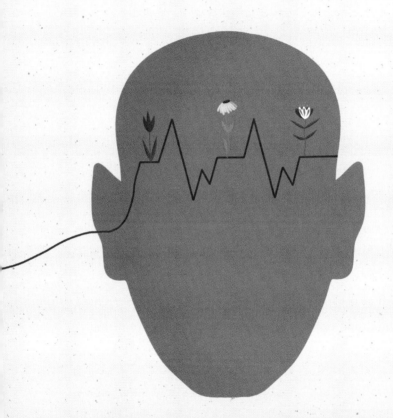

& listening heals

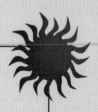

Struggle

Struggle. Why is struggle so hard to talk about? We've all gotten so used to seeing the polished lives of others, the snippets of light and laughter, the glamour and opulence, the perfect spouse and genius-children in harmony, the six-figure brand deals, work-free Tuesday afternoons, perfect teeth and everything in between ... so all that glitters must surely be gold, right?

No wonder we find it hard to talk about. In a sea of overnight success stories, 18-year-old self-made millionaires and mother-of-the-year awards being handed out left, right and centre, how are you supposed to say 'I need help'? How are you supposed to be vulnerable and human? Surely, you're going to be the only one, and is it even legal to admit that you're finding life difficult anymore?

When all you see is the highlights, it's hard to imagine that those stories are littered with lowlights, but the truth is, they are. Nobody lives on Cloud 9, we are merely brief visitors. Every person on this planet has hard days, bruises and bumps, grey phases, doubts, worries and the rest. So even though it can feel like struggle is a table for one, you are never alone, even if the other diners don't ever let it be known that they're also browsing the menu.

Through adversity, resilience is born. Struggle often arrives unannounced, uninvited and unyielding. It takes various forms, testing our limits, shaking the foundations of our being and pushing us to confront our fears and limitations. It is in these moments of struggle that we are granted the chance to truly understand our inner strength and capacity for growth.

So ask for help, ask for it boldly and honestly. There is strength in fighting for yourself, there is bravery in being vulnerable, and there is beauty in being human.

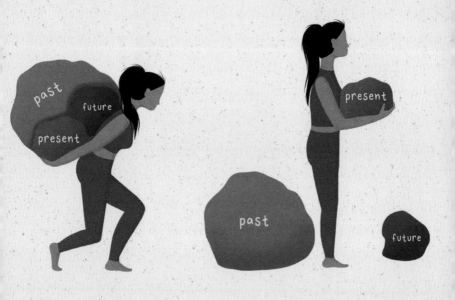

When it all gets too heavy, it's okay to put it down

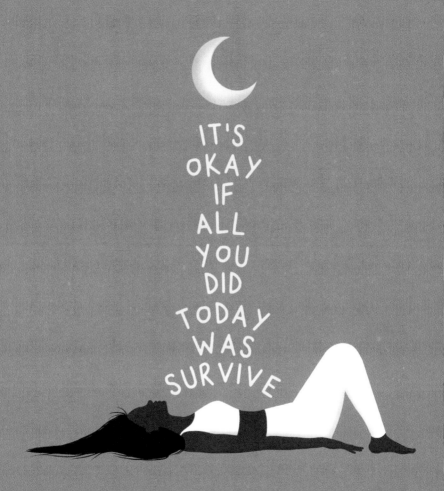

IT'S
OKAY
IF
ALL
YOU
DID
TODAY
WAS
SURVIVE

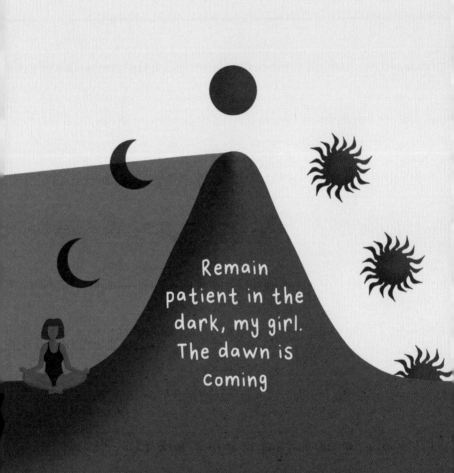

Remain patient in the dark, my girl. The dawn is coming

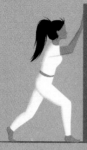

How it feels today

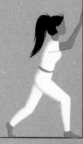

How it feels next week

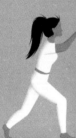

How it feels next month

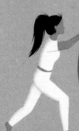

How it feels next year

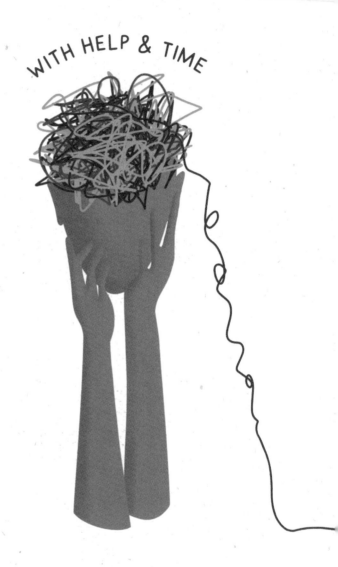

WITH HELP & TIME

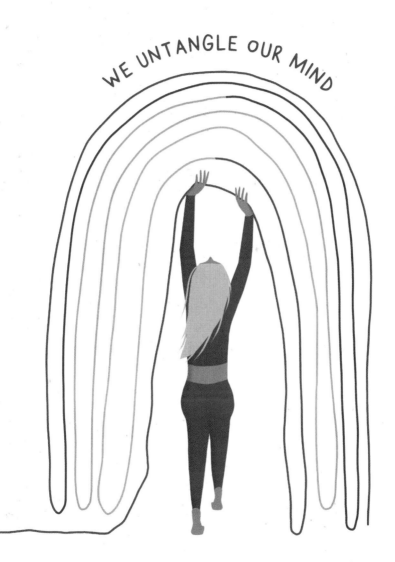

WE UNTANGLE OUR MIND

Struggle can feel like the loneliest place

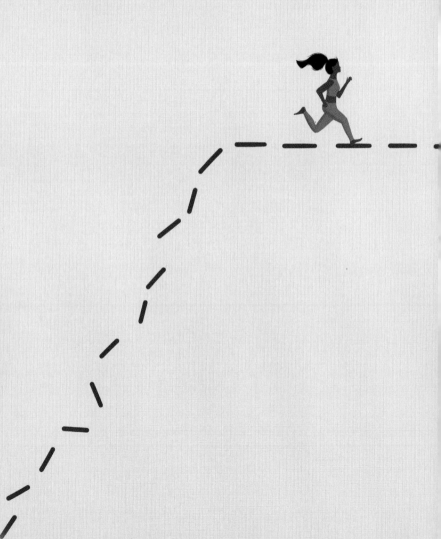

but you are never alone

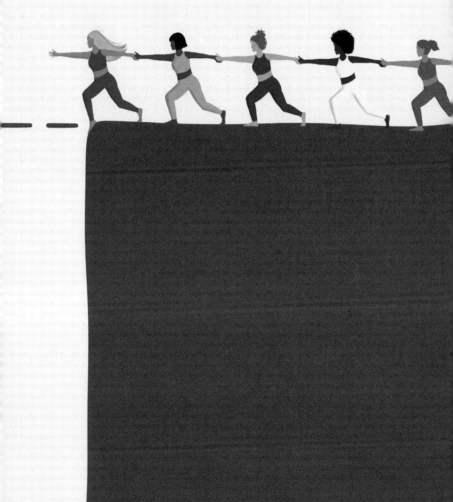

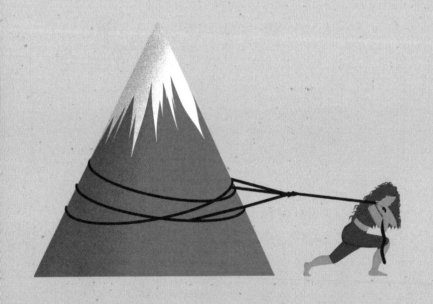

TRYING TO DO EVERYTHING AT ONCE

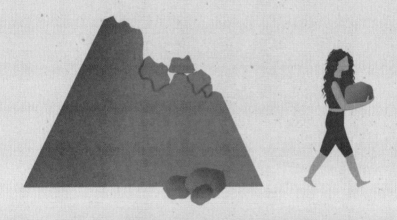

VS DOING A LITTLE EVERY DAY

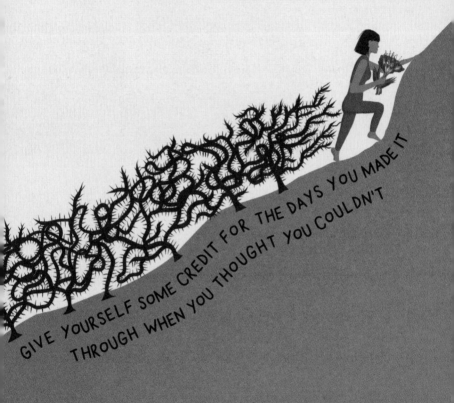

GIVE YOURSELF SOME CREDIT FOR THE DAYS YOU MADE IT THROUGH WHEN YOU THOUGHT YOU COULDN'T

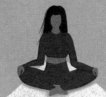

What people see

What someone is actually
going through

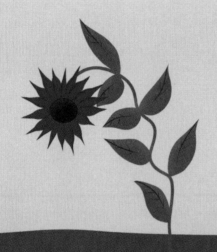

TRYING TO DO IT ALL ALONE CAN GET HEAVY

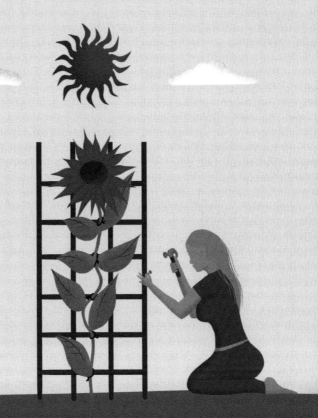

IT'S BETTER TO ACCEPT HELP AND SUPPORT

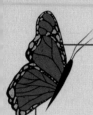

Self-love

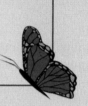

It's taken us a while, but we've finally got here. And by here, I mean a place where we are starting to understand and value the importance of self-love. I feel lucky to have been born into an era where it's no longer some taboo subject we back away from in the fear that we are seen as selfish.

Self-love isn't selfish. In fact, it's like filling up your own cup so much that you've got extra to share with others. Imagine if we all did it, how much there'd be to go around! It's like the energy booster that lets you be a more patient parent, a more present partner and a more attentive friend. When you treat yourself like you matter, it's like you're giving the universe permission to treat you that way too.

Try to imagine you've got this mental garden and self-love is the sunshine and water that makes your personal blooms thrive. It's not about being narcissistic or ignoring your flaws - it's about embracing the whole package, from the pretty petals we admire, to the mucky soil that nourishes from beneath. It's realising that you're worthy of care and kindness, just as you are.

Self-love is about saying 'no' when you need to, setting boundaries that protect your energy, and giving yourself permission to prioritise your own well-being. It's like being your own BFF, someone who's got your back no matter what. It's taking the time to check in with yourself, like you would with a friend. How are you feeling today? What do you need?

We live in a world that's quick to point out what's 'wrong' with us, making self-love a bit of a rebel act. It's the audacity to stand up and say, 'Hey, I'm imperfect, but I'm worthy of love and effort.' It's about silencing that inner critic and replacing those negative thoughts with words that lift you up instead of tearing you down.

Let's unravel the layers, challenge the misconceptions, and embrace the journey of learning to love ourselves a little more each day. Because you, my lovely, deserve all the love, care and kindness that you so freely give to others. It's time to sprinkle some of that magic right back where it belongs: on yourself.

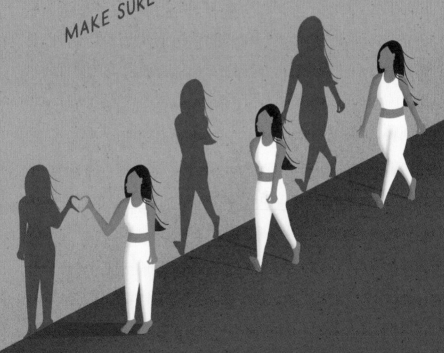

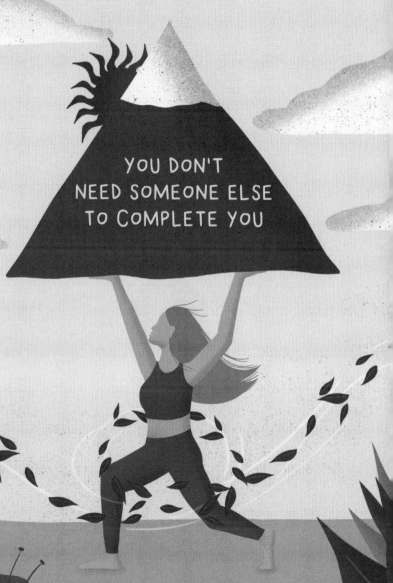

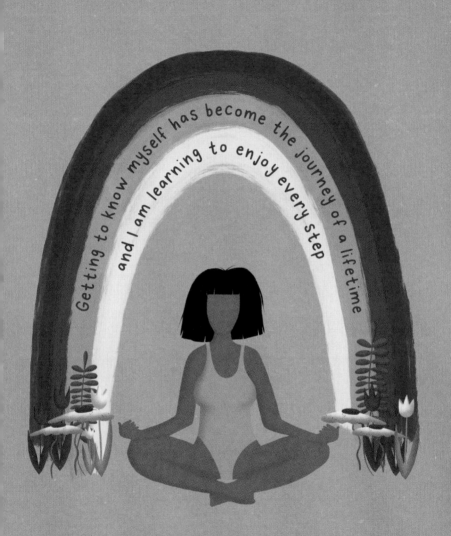

Getting to know myself has become the journey of a lifetime and I am learning to enjoy every step

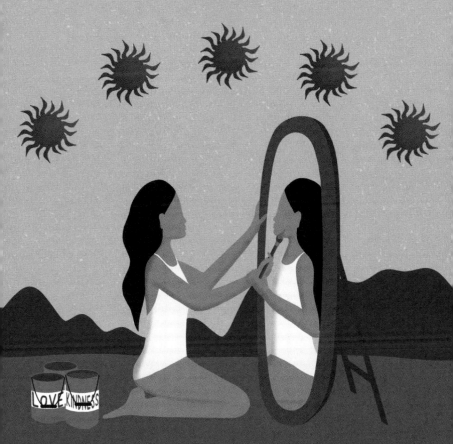

You are the greatest project
you'll ever work on

Dear self,

I know some days
the staircase feels
very steep and like
you'll never take
the next step, but
you're doing the
best you can, and
for that, I just
want to say I'm
proud of you.
Keep going.

Love, me x

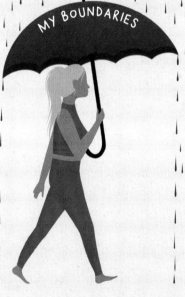

SELF-CRITICISM

TOXIC PEOPLE

COMPARISON

GUILT

OVERWORKING

MY BOUNDARIES

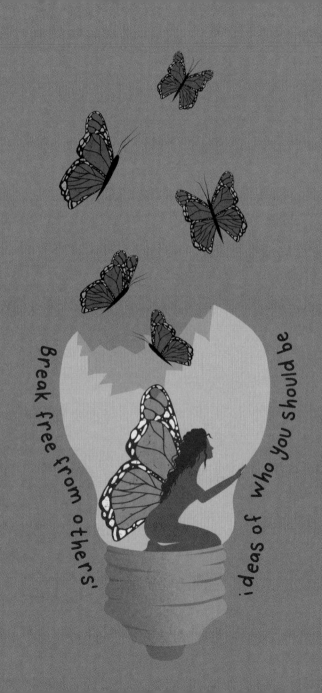

Break free from others' ideas of who you should be

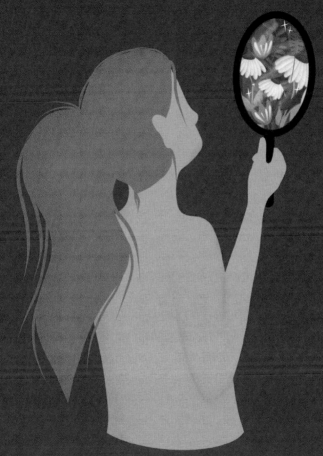

See your beauty

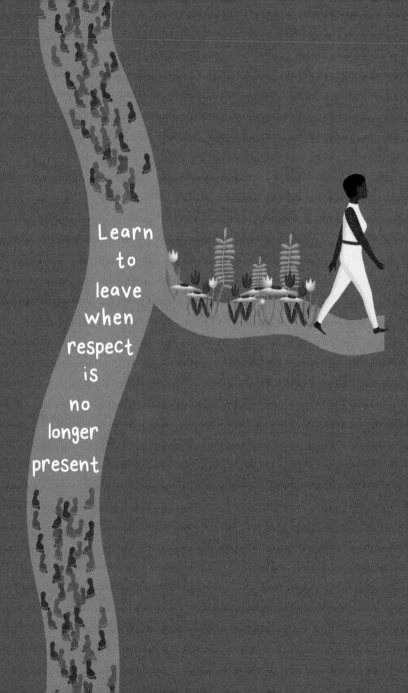

Learn to leave when respect is no longer present

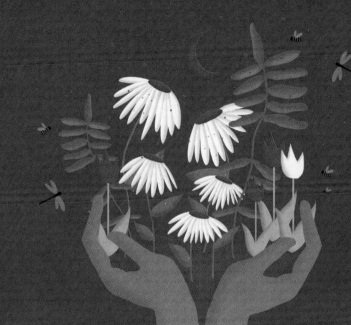

DON'T HIDE YOUR MAGIC

WHAT A BEAUTIFUL THING IT IS

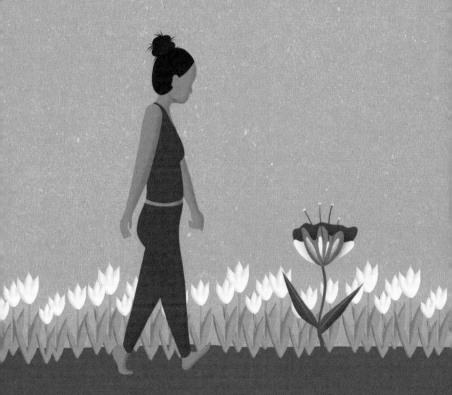

TO BE DIFFERENT

Today, I choose me

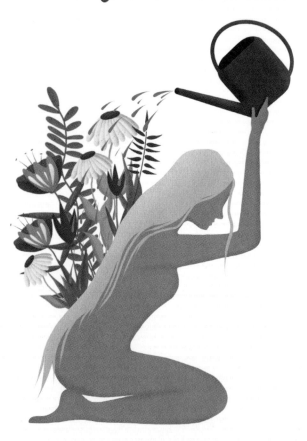

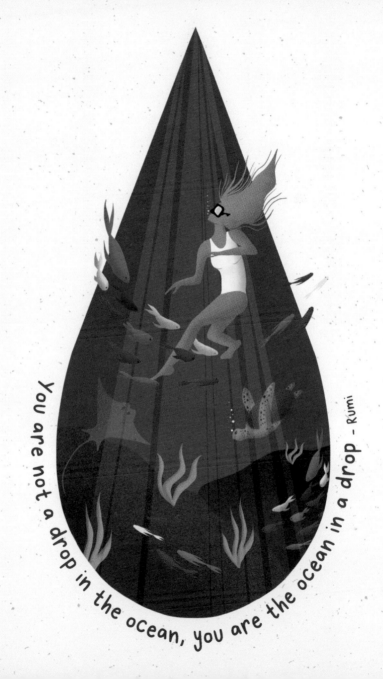

You are not a drop in the ocean, you are the ocean in a drop. – Rumi

DON'T COMPARE YOUR FIRST CHAPTER

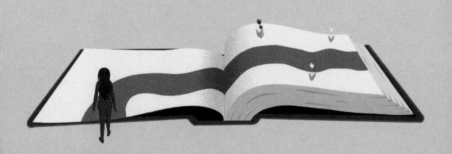

TO SOMEONE ELSE'S TENTH CHAPTER

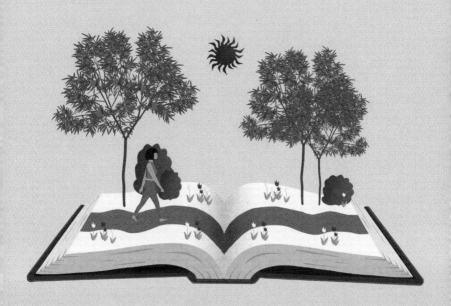

Empowerment

Empowerment feels like such a mighty thing, something we may not believe ourselves to be worthy of. It can feel like something reserved for those who create big change in the world, those who stand tall against adversity, carry signs at big political protests, give speeches on world platforms, you know, the Greta Thunbergs and Malala Yousafzais of the world. But then I think of my 5-year-old self dancing to songs by the Spice Girls in the height of the 'girl power' movement of the 90s and I remember that feeling, that feeling of 'I can do anything', all the while flexing my muscles in the mirror, stood in my mum's high heels. That was empowerment, right there in my childhood bedroom with no UN podium in sight. Just a girl and a song.

The truth is, empowerment quietly lurks in all of our day-to-day lives, just waiting for its moment.

In a world that may sometimes try to shrink us, empowerment is the act of expansion. It's about breaking free from the chains of self-doubt and societal constraints, about rewriting the narratives that have told us we're too small or too insignificant. It's in those moments when we dare to step out of the shadows, when we lift our heads and say, 'I matter, and my story matters'.

Empowerment isn't about being impervious to challenges - it's about having the courage to face them head-on. It's the quiet resilience that fuels us when the road ahead seems steep and daunting. Just as a single candle can pierce through the darkness, our empowered selves have the ability to illuminate even the dimmest corners of our lives.

So, let's challenge the notion that empowerment is reserved for the extraordinary. Let's celebrate the small victories, the daily triumphs over self-doubt and the subtle ways we reclaim control over our lives.

Let's remember that each step taken towards empowerment ripples outwards, creating waves of change not only within ourselves but also in the lives of those who witness our transformation.

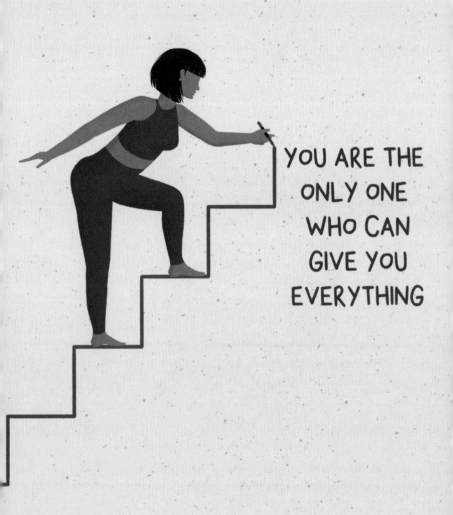

YOU ARE THE
ONLY ONE
WHO CAN
GIVE YOU
EVERYTHING

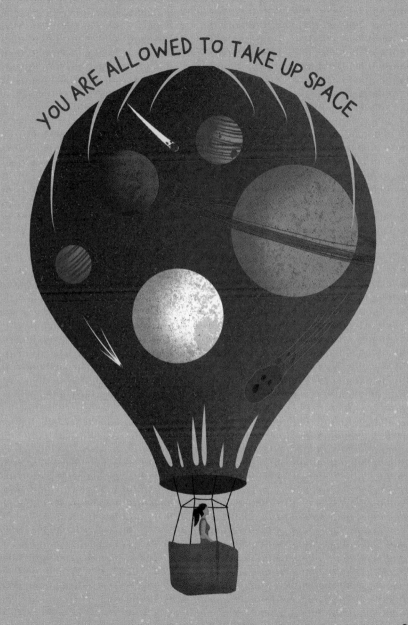

You have within you everything you need

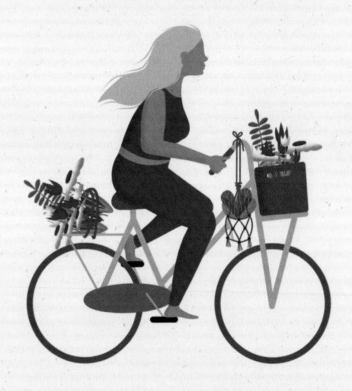

to get to where you want to go

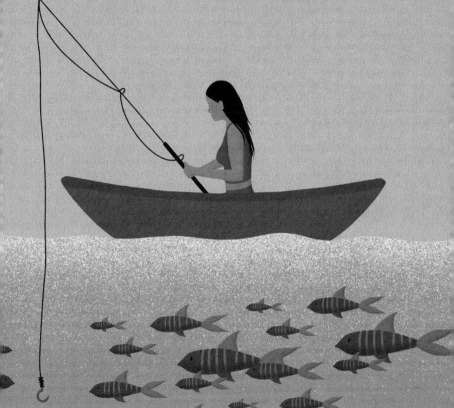

YOUR PATIENCE IS YOUR POWER

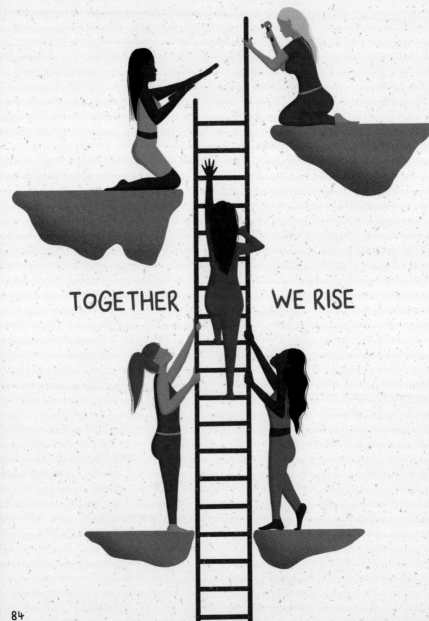

TOGETHER   WE RISE

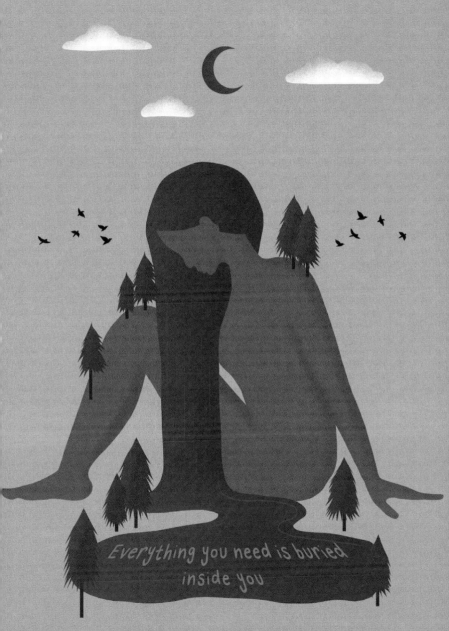

Everything you need is buried inside you

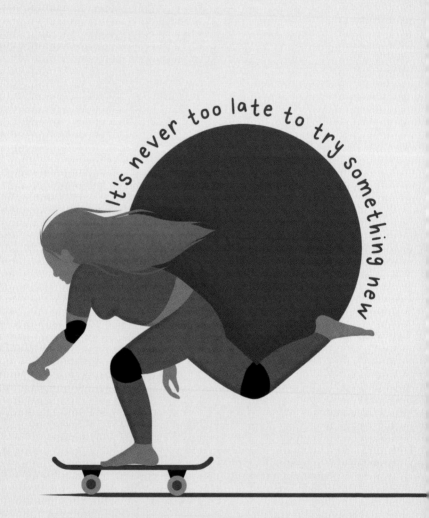

It's never too late to try something new

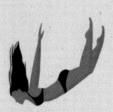
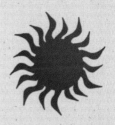
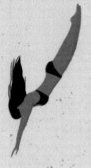

SHE BELIEVED SHE COULD, SO SHE DID

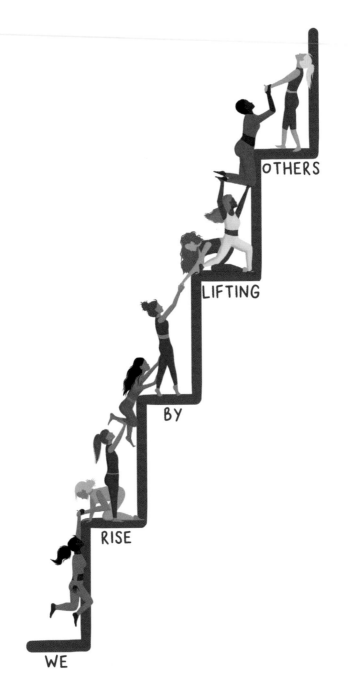

OTHERS

LIFTING

BY

RISE

WE

DON'T YOU EVER LET SOMEONE ELSE DECIDE WHAT YOU CAN ACHIEVE, MY GIRL

YOU CAN'T DO IT. YOU CAN'T DO IT.

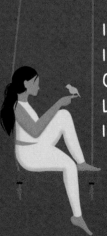

IF
IT
COMES,
LET
IT

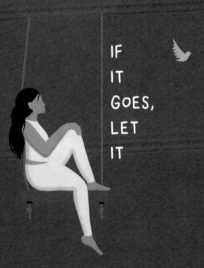

IF
IT
GOES,
LET
IT

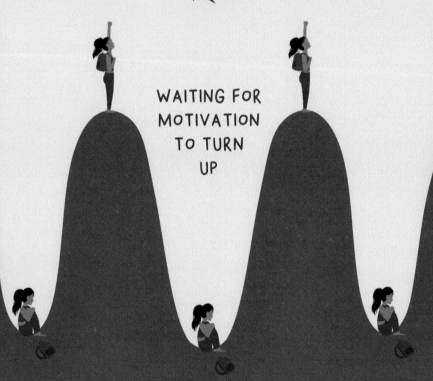

WAITING FOR
MOTIVATION
TO TURN
UP

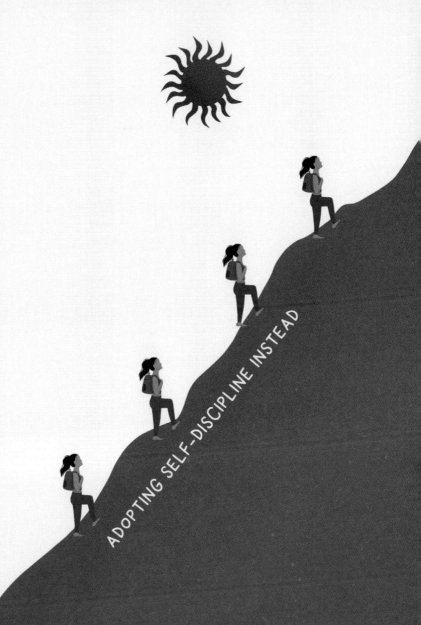

ADOPTING SELF-DISCIPLINE INSTEAD

Progress

Progress is like the journey of a thousand miles, but instead of giant leaps, it's all about those tiny, relentless steps you take every single day. Sometimes it feels like we need hard evidence of our progress, like racking up followers on social media or winning an award for an accomplishment, but really, progress sits much more subtly in our daily lives. It's the 'aha!' moment when you learn something new, and the satisfying feeling of crossing things off your to-do list.

It can be so subtle, it's hard to see sometimes. I like to 'zoom out' on my year and look at the differences made between this year and last; that's where you really see all those tiny pieces of the puzzle come together.

And progress isn't about speed; if you need to 'zoom out' on your last two or three years, that's also okay! Progress doesn't mean you have to sprint all the time.

It's not about racing through life like a maniac.
It's about finding your own pace, recognising that
sometimes you take big strides and other times you
take baby steps, and that's perfectly okay.

In a world that can feel like a highlight reel of other
people's achievements, progress is a gentle reminder
that your journey is your own. It's about realising
that comparison is a slippery slope to nowhere and
that your path, with all its twists and turns, is
unique and beautiful.

Progress isn't just about reaching the finish line; it's
about enjoying the scenic route. It's the realisation
that sometimes the detours, the wrong turns
and the unexpected pit stops are where the most
exciting adventures happen. It's about celebrating
the process as much as the outcome.

So, as we embark on this thrilling expedition into
the land of progress, let's do it with the spirit of
an explorer. Let's embrace the ups and downs, the
triumphs and the setbacks, and let's remember
that the journey itself is where the real magic
happens. Because, my friend, progress isn't just about
reaching a destination; it's about embracing the joy
of the ride and the incredible growth that happens
along the way.

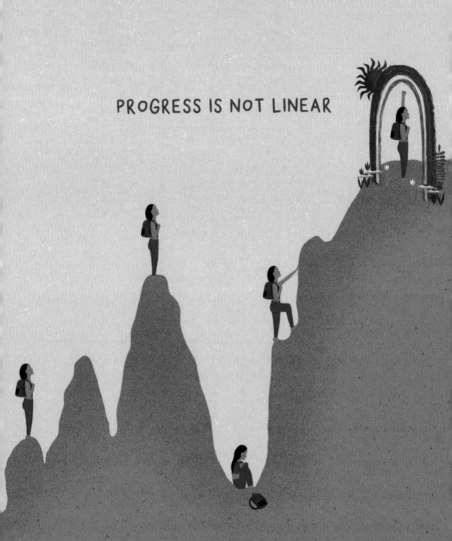

PROGRESS IS NOT LINEAR

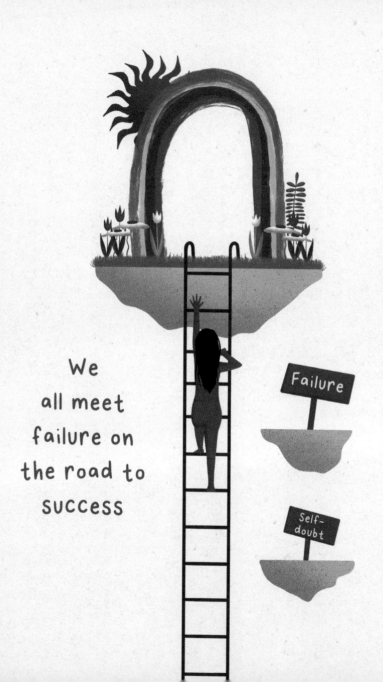

We all meet failure on the road to success

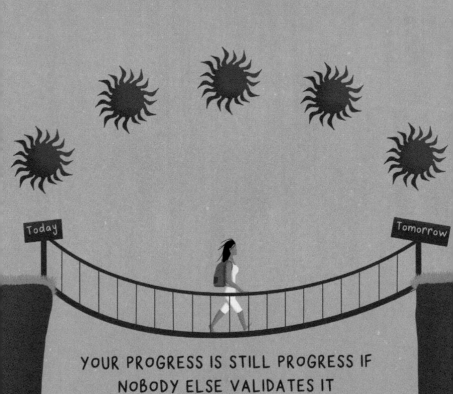

YOUR PROGRESS IS STILL PROGRESS IF
NOBODY ELSE VALIDATES IT

Recharge yourself & marvel at the energy you create

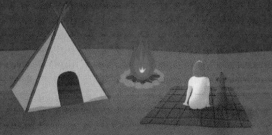

I HAVEN'T FAILED.

I'VE JUST FOUND 10,000 WAYS THAT DIDN'T WORK

- Thomas Edison

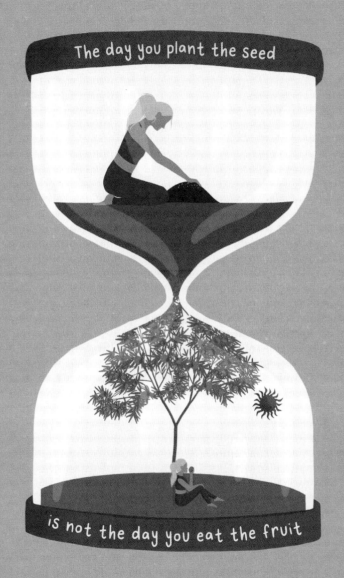

The day you plant the seed

is not the day you eat the fruit

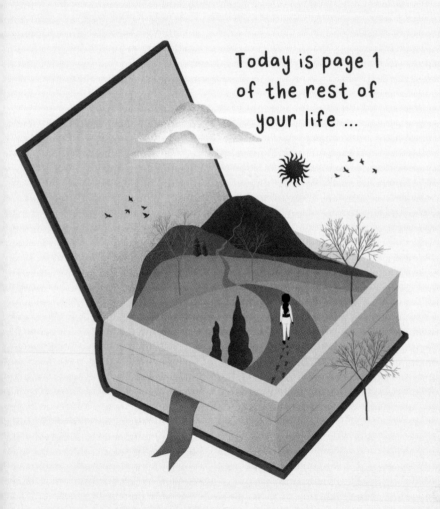

Today is page 1
of the rest of
your life ...

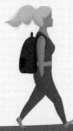

Today's progress felt like this

This year's progress actually looks like this

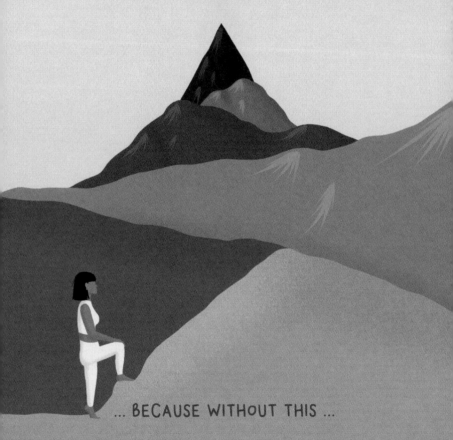

I PROMISE TO HONOUR MY PROGRESS
THROUGHOUT EVERY STEP OF THIS
JOURNEY...

... BECAUSE WITHOUT THIS ...

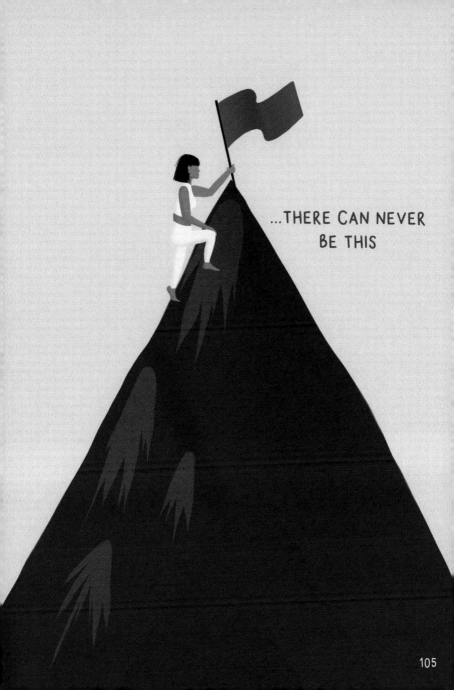

...THERE CAN NEVER
BE THIS

Our direction forward is more important than our speed

SOMETIMES
YOU NEED
TO WEIGH
THE FEAR
OF THE
JUMP
AGAINST
THE FEAR
OF NEVER
KNOWING

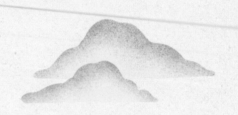

IF YOU DO WHAT YOU DID,
YOU GET WHAT YOU GOT...

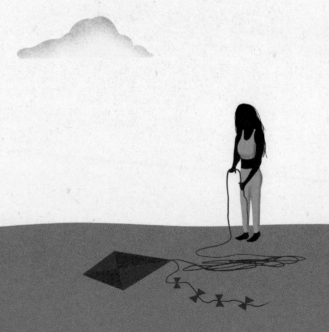

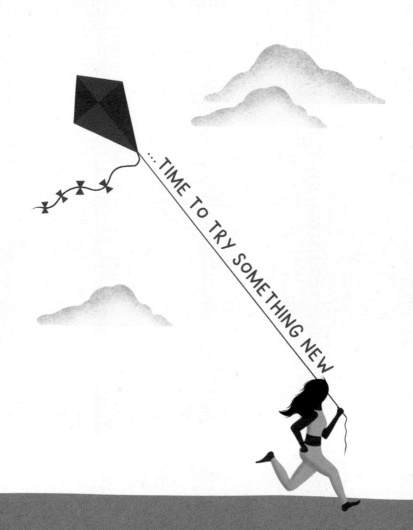

... TIME TO TRY SOMETHING NEW

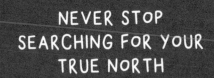

NEVER STOP
SEARCHING FOR YOUR
TRUE NORTH

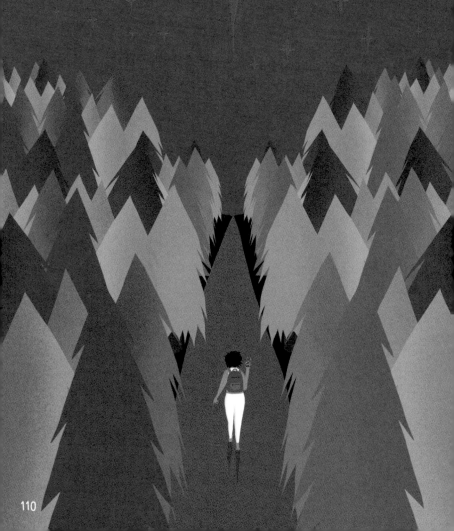

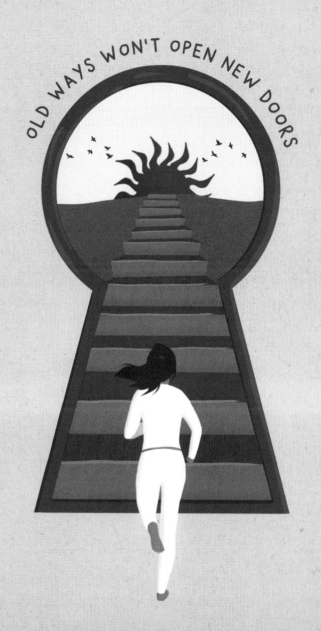

OLD WAYS WON'T OPEN NEW DOORS

111

Acceptance

Acceptance and growth go hand-in-hand. At first glance, acceptance sounds weak, like you're rolling over and taking everything that happens to you. But oh my lovely, acceptance is so much more than that!

It comes in so many shapes and sizes. From accepting yourself for who you are and embracing all the things that make you, you, flaws and all. To accepting situations as they happened and moving on from them, understanding that you cannot change them. It could be that you learn to accept other people as they are, or that you accept your failures as part of your progress.

It's like life is a river, and you're in a canoe. You can paddle against the current, cursing every bump and twist in the water, or you can relax, let go of the oars and float downstream. That's acceptance in a nutshell - it's choosing the latter, embracing the ebb and flow of existence.

Now, it's crucial to understand that acceptance isn't about resignation. It's not waving the white flag to life's challenges; it's acknowledging that some things are beyond our control. It's like realising you can't change the weather, but you can choose your outfit for the day.

Acceptance doesn't mean you stop growing or improving. It's not about complacency; it's about making friends with the present moment. It's the realisation that, despite the chaos and imperfections, you're okay right here, right now.

It's time for us to explore how accepting the reality of who you are, where you've been, and where you're going can set you free. It's time to let go of resistance and let acceptance be your compass on this wild journey.

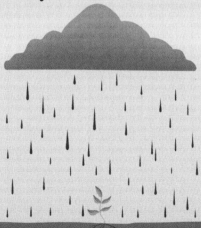

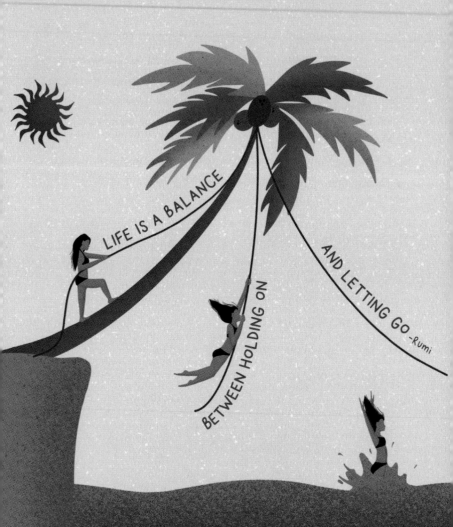

LIFE IS A BALANCE

BETWEEN HOLDING ON

AND LETTING GO -Rumi

THE PAST HAPPENED

THAT I CANNOT CHANGE

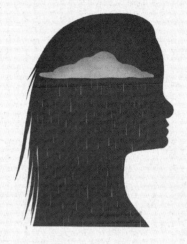

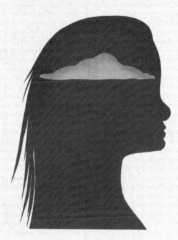

I ACCEPT IT

BUT I WON'T LET IT
STEAL TODAY

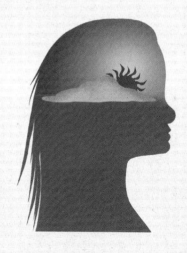

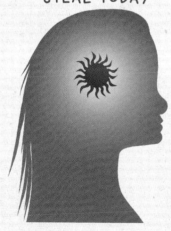

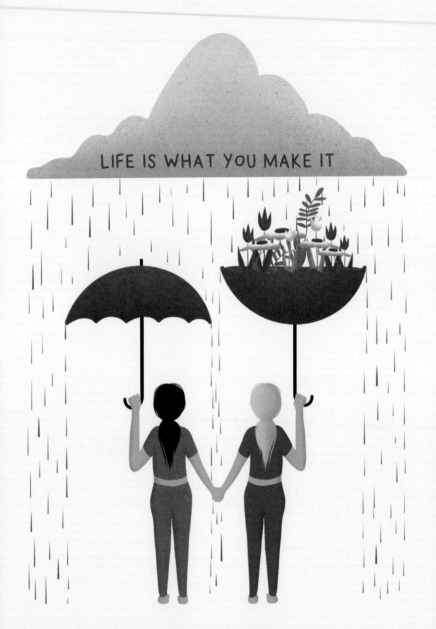

LIFE IS WHAT YOU MAKE IT

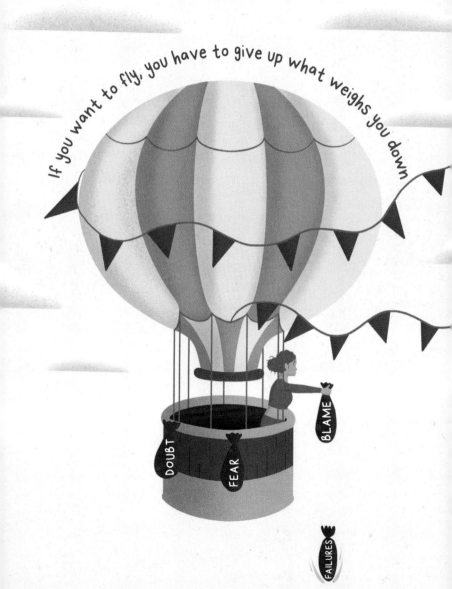

If you want to fly, you have to give up what weighs you down

DOUBT

FEAR

BLAME

FAILURES

WHO THEY WANT
ME TO BE

WHO I REALLY
AM

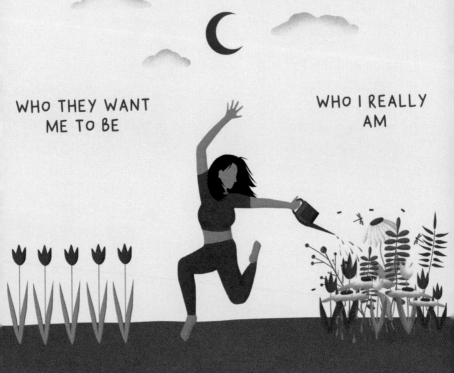

ACCEPT FAILURE AS PART OF THE PROCESS

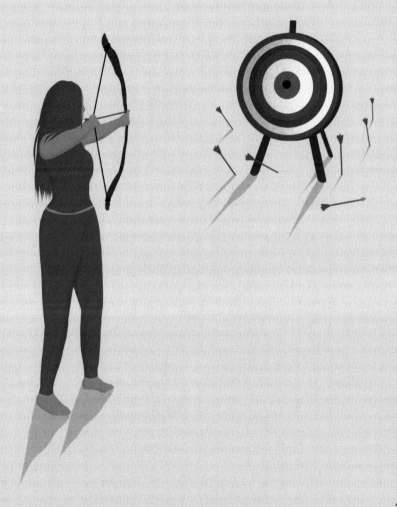

You can only move on

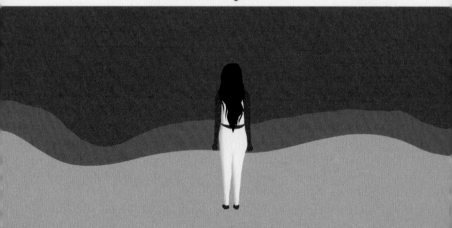

once you accept it's over

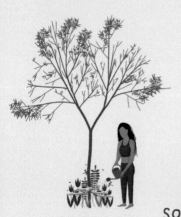

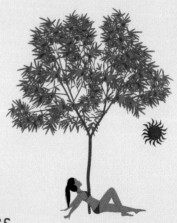

SOME THINGS
HAVE
TO END FOR
BETTER THINGS
TO BEGIN

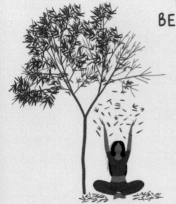

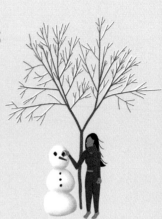

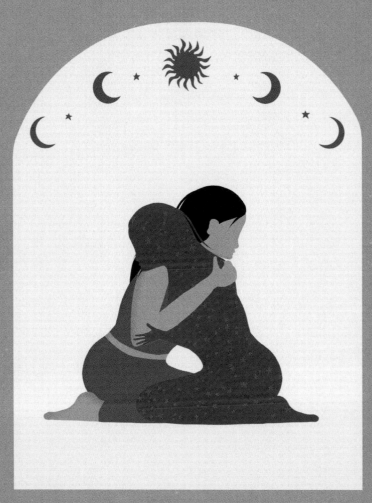

STOP FIGHTING WHO YOU ARE AND ACCEPT HER
MIND, BODY AND SOUL

No rain

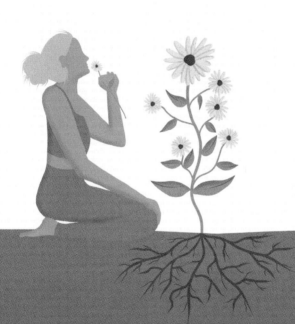

No flowers

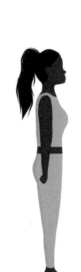

Their
success
is
not
your
failure

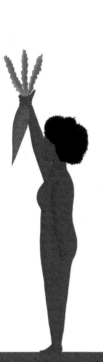

I am worthy of this journey

Focus

Focus. Why is it so important that there's a whole chapter dedicated to it? It's that secret ingredient that turns a scatterbrained day into a productive one, that helps you dive deep into what truly matters, and keeps you from getting lost in the whirlwind of distractions.

In a world that's constantly buzzing with notifications, texts, and all sorts of digital tugs, maintaining focus can feel like trying to balance on a unicycle during an earthquake. It's about navigating a minefield of interruptions and staying on course, even when everything around you is vying for your attention.

Focus isn't just about honing in on a single task - it's also about finding clarity amidst the noise. It's like tuning your radio dial to the right station when all you've been hearing is static. It's about carving out moments of stillness and mental clarity in a world that often feels like a whirlwind. Focusing on the things that matter most and dodging those marketing landmines, which would have you believe that bigger houses, faster cars and more labels is what you should focus on. That's what's important here.

Focus isn't about shutting everything out. It's about being present, about immersing yourself fully in the task at hand. Whether that be time with your loved ones, disconnecting in nature or working on your passion project. It's like finding that sweet spot where time seems to stand still, and all that matters is the here and now. I truly believe that focus and consistency are the ingredients to success.

So, let's take a minute to really understand the value of focus and the skill it takes to stay true to your path. Because in a world that's constantly pulling us in a million directions, the ability to focus is a superpower that lets us carve our own path, one intentional step at a time.

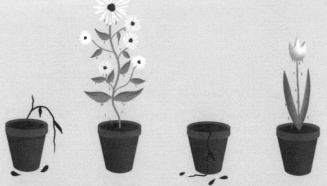

I AM FOCUSED ON MY OWN JOURNEY, ON MY OWN STORY. No ONE ELSE'S, JUST MINE

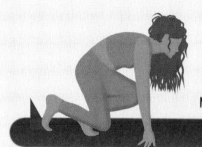

RESTART AND REFOCUS AS MANY TIMES AS YOU NEED TO

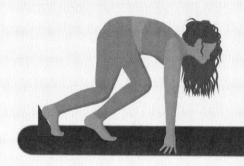

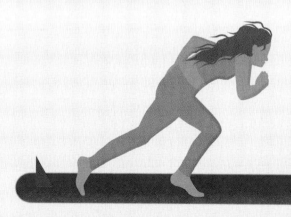

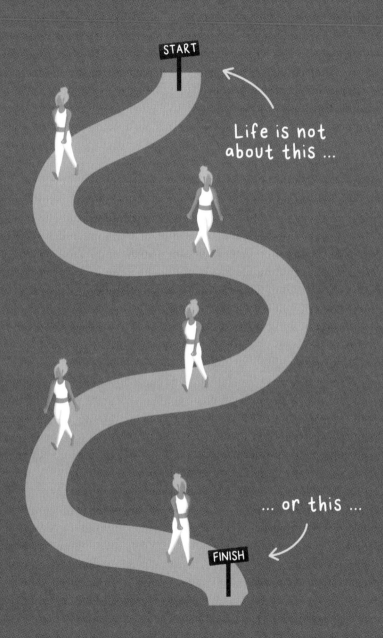

START

Life is not
about this ...

... or this ...

FINISH

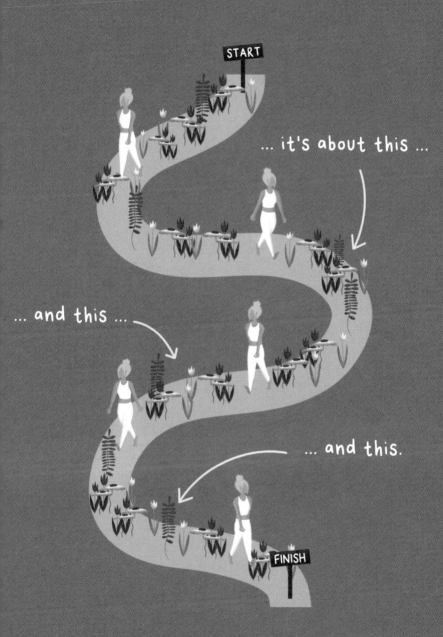

START

... it's about this ...

... and this ...

... and this.

FINISH

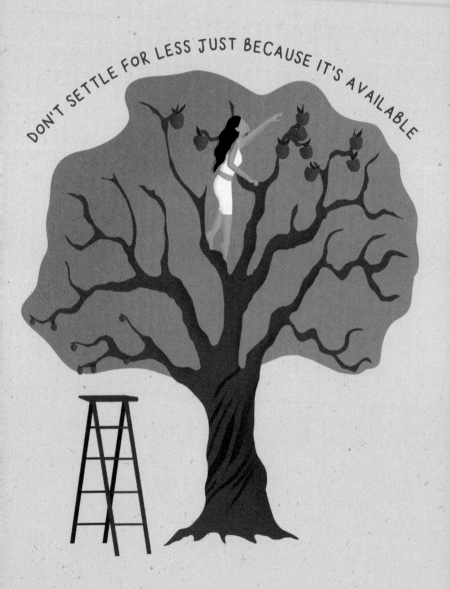

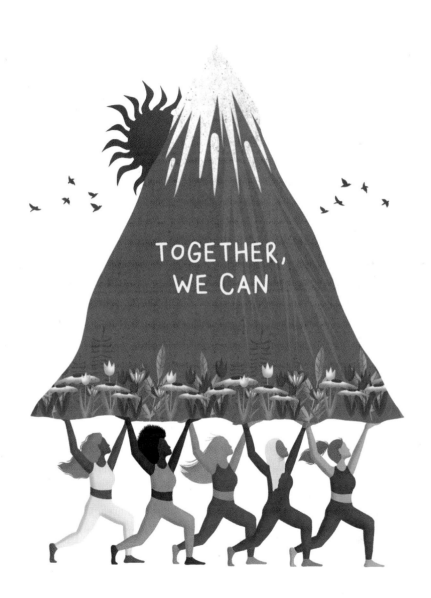

Just keep showing up when everyone else quits

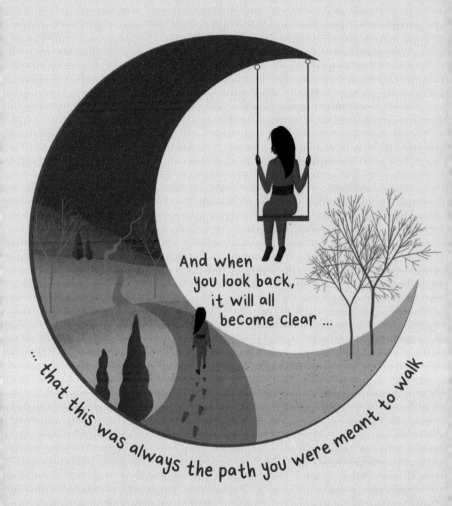

And when
you look back,
it will all
become clear ...

... that this was always the path you were meant to walk

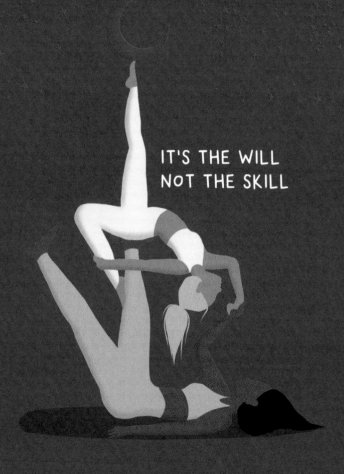

IT'S THE WILL
NOT THE SKILL

FOCUS ON WHAT REALLY MATTERS

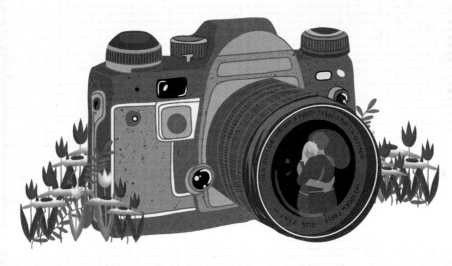

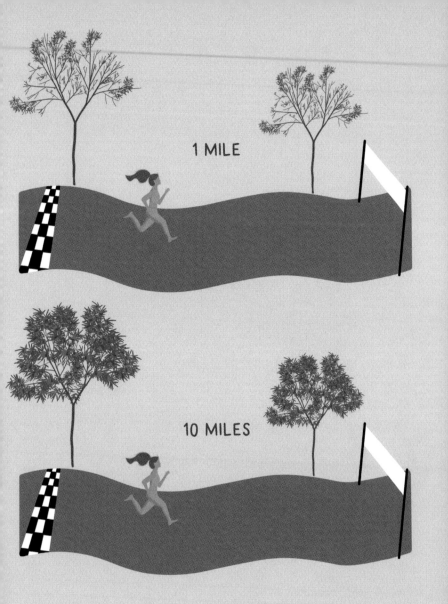

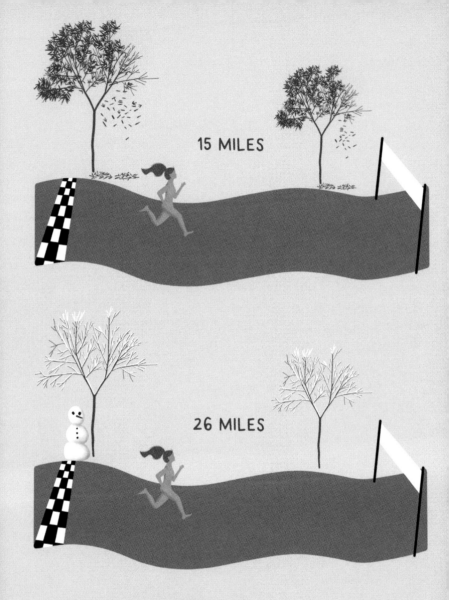

15 MILES

26 MILES

PROGRESS TAKES TIME

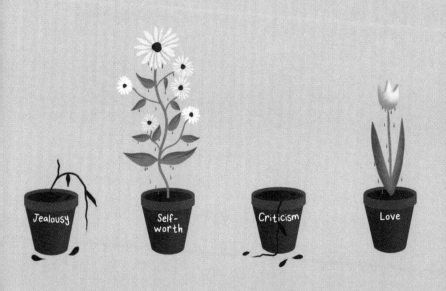

What you give energy to ...

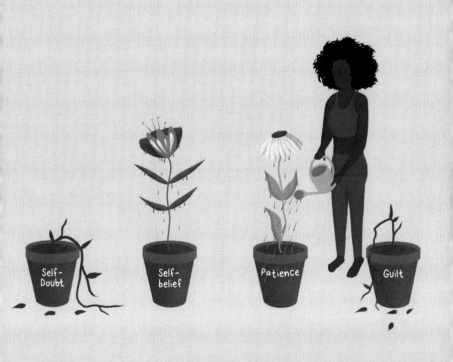

... grows

Self-care

Self-care, oh, even the words make me feel warm and cosy. It's like the soothing balm for your tired soul, the life jacket that keeps you afloat in the sea of chaos, and the secure embrace you give yourself when the world feels like a whirlwind.

Now, let's clear something up. Self-care isn't selfish. Repeat after me: it's NoT selfish! In fact, it's the exact opposite. When you take the time to look after yourself, you're actually supercharging your ability to give back to others. It's like that airplane safety demo - you gotta put on your oxygen mask first before assisting others.

And let's bust a myth: self-care isn't always about extravagant spa days or exotic vacations (though those are fabulous too). It's about the everyday rituals that nourish your mind, body and soul.

It's the moments you steal for yourself, whether it's reading a book, taking a long walk or simply savouring a piece of chocolate without guilt.

Self-care is also about setting boundaries. It's like building a fence around your emotional garden to protect your precious blooms from trampling feet. It's about knowing when to say no, when to step back, and when to prioritise your own well-being.

Taking care of yourself isn't just a luxury; it's a necessity. It's like a love letter you write to yourself every day, a reminder that you are worthy of care, rest, and all the good things in life.

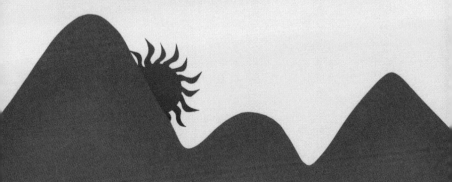

CHOOSE WISELY WHERE TO SPEND YOUR ENERGY

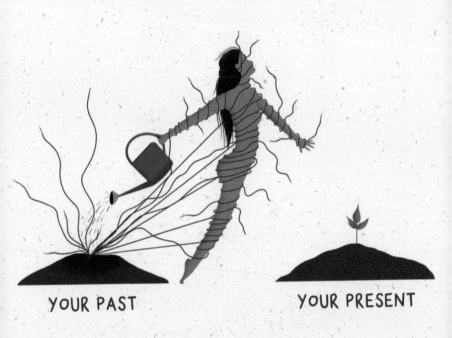

YOUR PAST

YOUR PRESENT

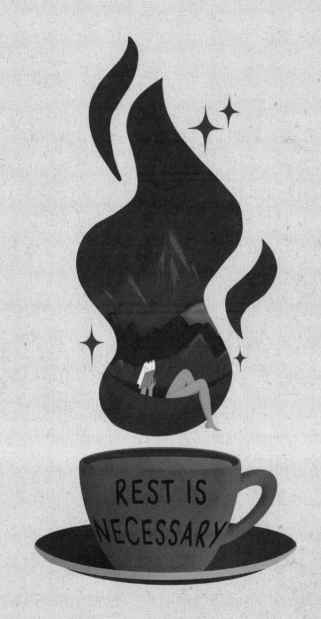

REST IS NECESSARY

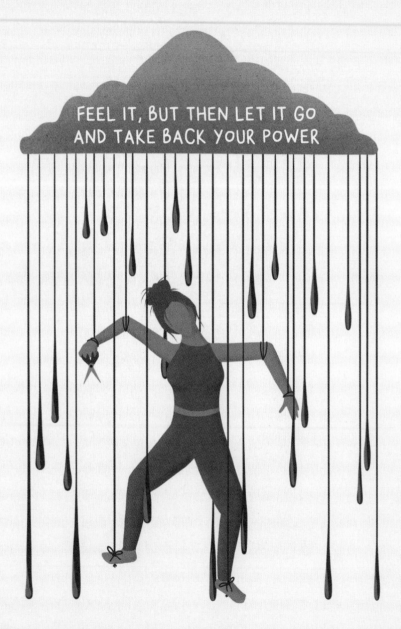

~~HUSTLE~~

BALANCE

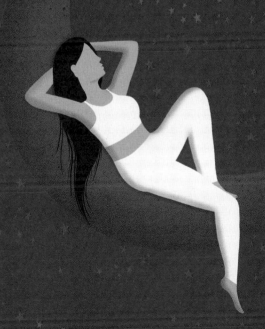

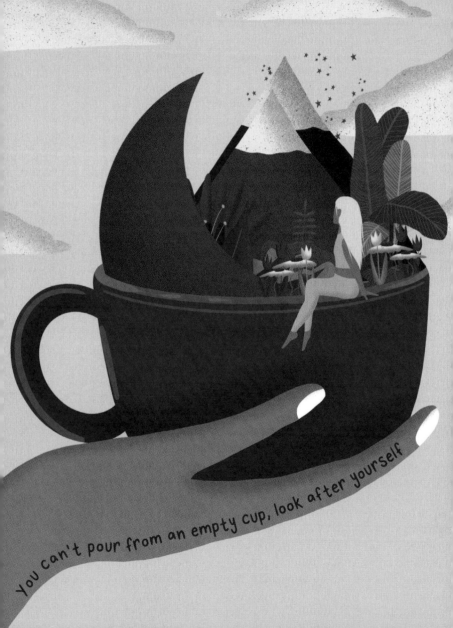

You can't pour from an empty cup, look after yourself

TRUST YOUR GUT

ENERGY DOESN'T LIE

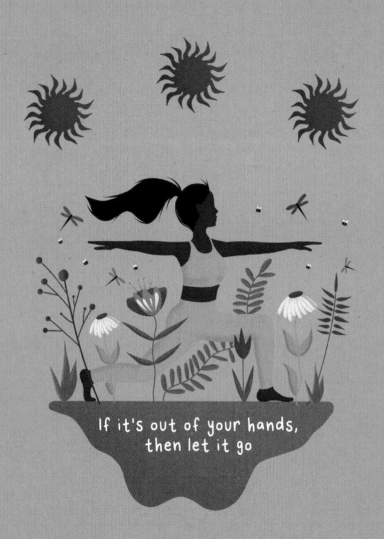

If it's out of your hands,
then let it go

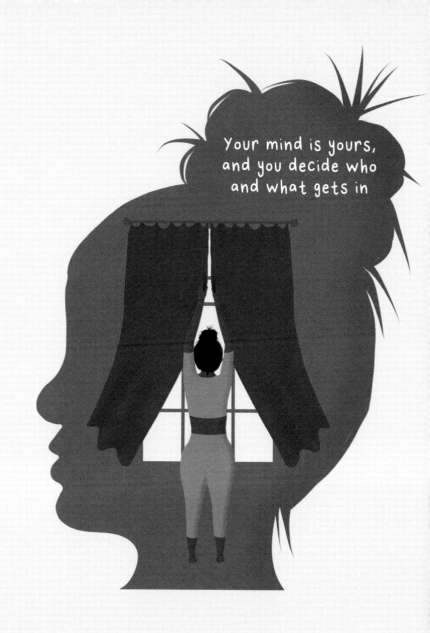

Your mind is yours, and you decide who and what gets in

I spotted a pattern ...

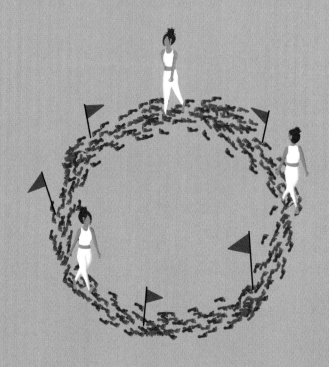

... so I decided to break free

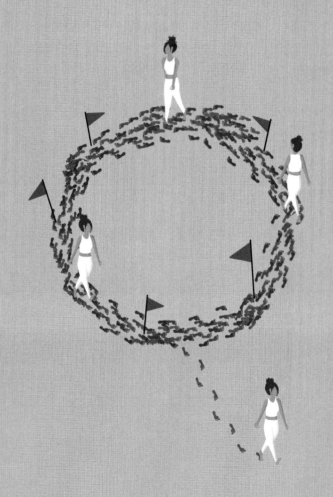

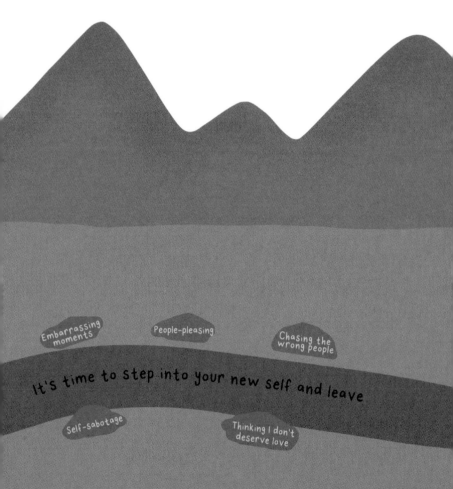

Embarrassing moments

People-pleasing

Chasing the wrong people

It's time to step into your new self and leave

Self-sabotage

Thinking I don't deserve love

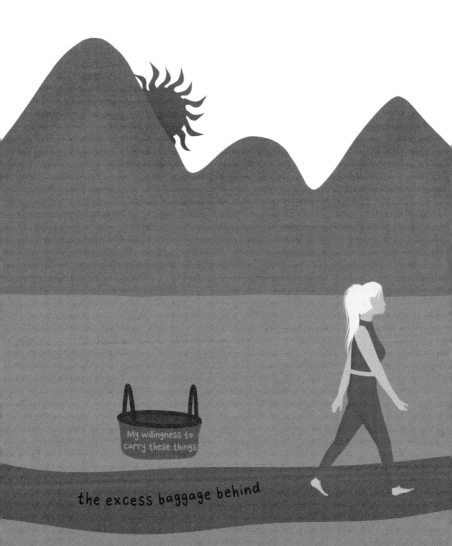

My willingness to
carry these things

the excess baggage behind

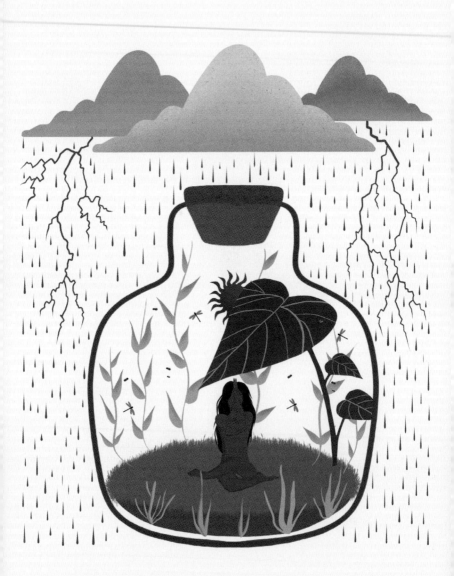

REST CAN BE REFUGE FROM THE STORM

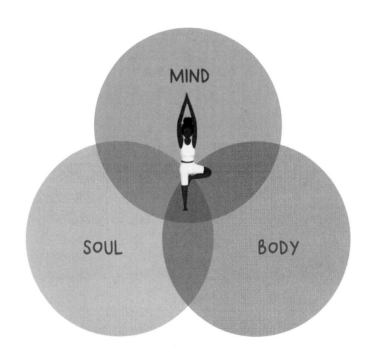

FIND YOURSELF IN

MIND

SOUL

BODY

HARMONY

Strength

What's the first thing that comes to mind when you read 'strength'? Was it a physical attribute, mental, behavioural or something completely different? I think most of us tend to subconsciously pair the word with muscular gym-regulars, people who would effortlessly scale a tree to save the neighbour's cat, or run half-marathons just for fun.

As I've gotten older, the word has revealed itself to carry many meanings. Physical strength is healthy and admirable, but mental strength? That's the stuff that gives me goosebumps. There's nothing on this planet more powerful than someone who has conquered their own mind.

But man, oh man, does it take some work to get there. And where even is 'there'? I don't really believe there is a final destination when it comes to working on yourself. Every person on this planet is a work in progress when it comes to strength, and it sure isn't linear. We have days where we carry our metaphorical baggage so easily we practically spin it on the tip of our fingers like a basketball, and other days, well, other days, it's so heavy it's like being buried by it.

Mental strength isn't about suppressing your emotions either. It's not about bottling up your feelings and pretending everything's peachy when it's not. It's about recognising your emotions, from the happy dances to the ugly cries, and finding healthy ways to deal with them. It's like giving yourself an emotional toolkit, complete with tools for tackling stress, anxiety and whatever else life tosses your way.

Let's explore what it means to build resilience, boost self-confidence, and handle whatever curveballs life throws at us. Because, my lovely, mental strength isn't about being invincible - it's about being beautifully, unapologetically human and showing up for your life with all the strength you've got.

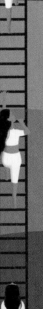

YOU

ARE

STRONGER

THAN

YOUR

HARDEST

DAYS

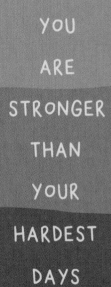

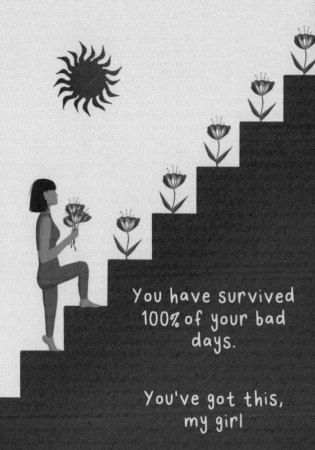

You have survived
100% of your bad
days.

You've got this,
my girl

163

Strength
is
pushing
yourself
to
your
limits

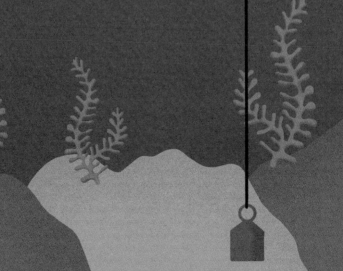

Strength
is
knowing
when
to
come
up
for
air

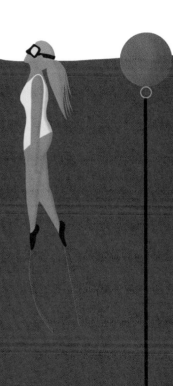

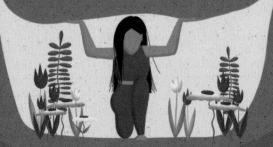

sometimes
you need to
meet
rock bottom
to find out just
how strong you are

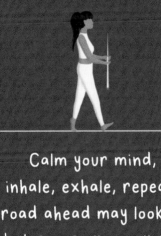

Calm your mind,
inhale, exhale, repeat.
The road ahead may look tough,
but so are you, my girl

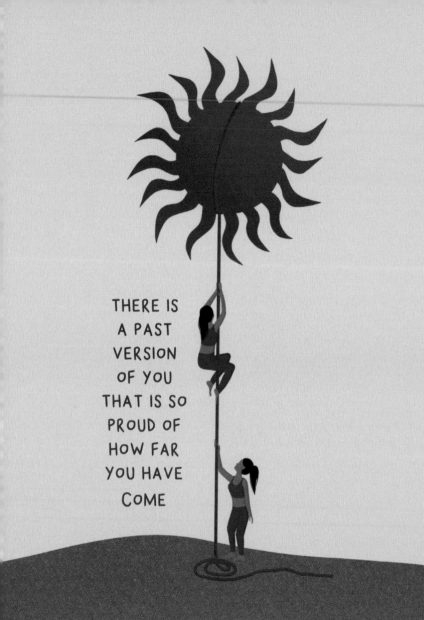

THERE IS
A PAST
VERSION
OF YOU
THAT IS SO
PROUD OF
HOW FAR
YOU HAVE
COME

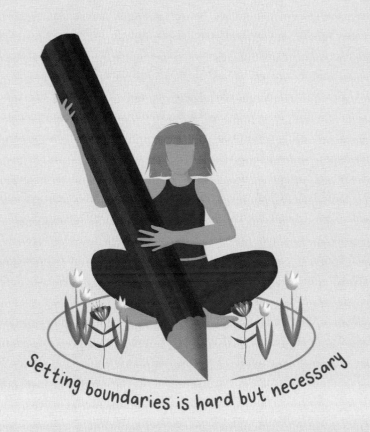

Setting boundaries is hard but necessary

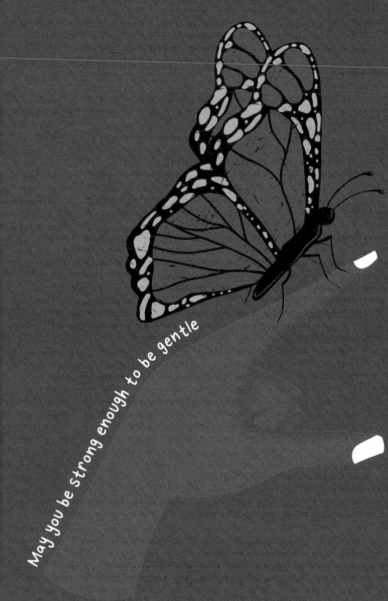

May you be strong enough to be gentle

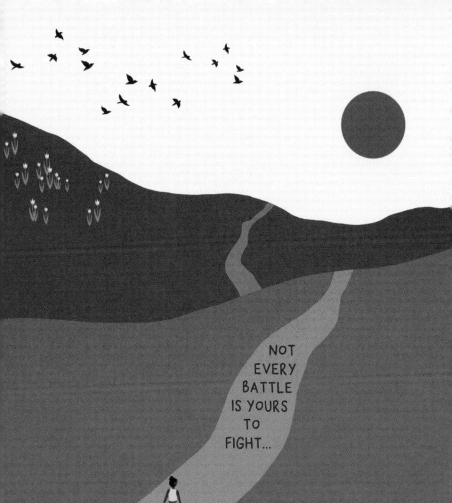

NOT EVERY BATTLE IS YOURS TO FIGHT...

...THERE IS STRENGTH IN WALKING AWAY

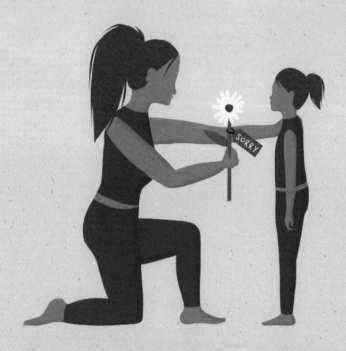

Accountability requires strength

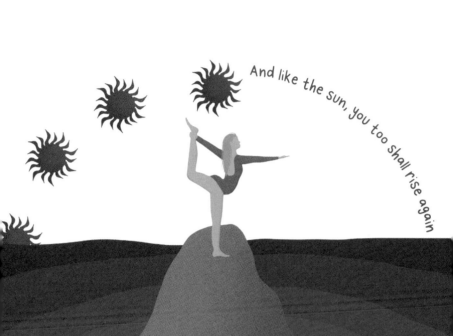

And like the sun, you too shall rise again

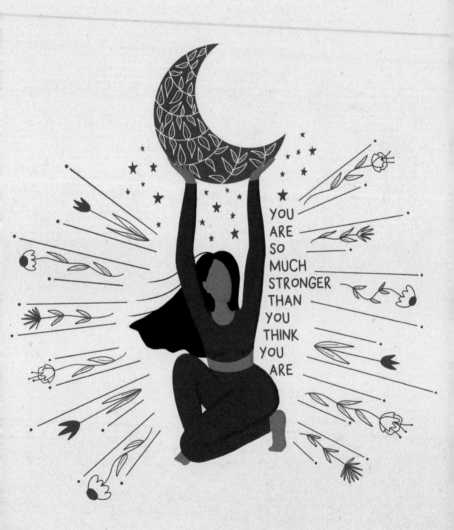

YOU
ARE
SO
MUCH
STRONGER
THAN
YOU
THINK
YOU
ARE

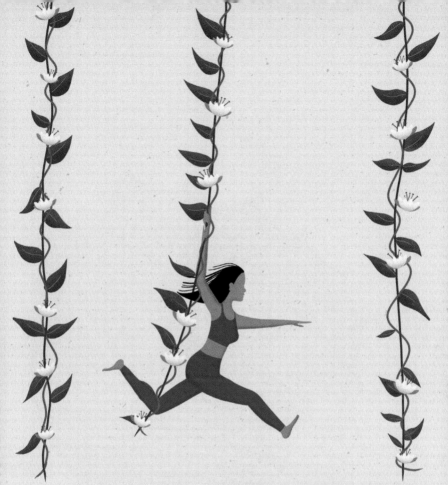

KEEP GOING

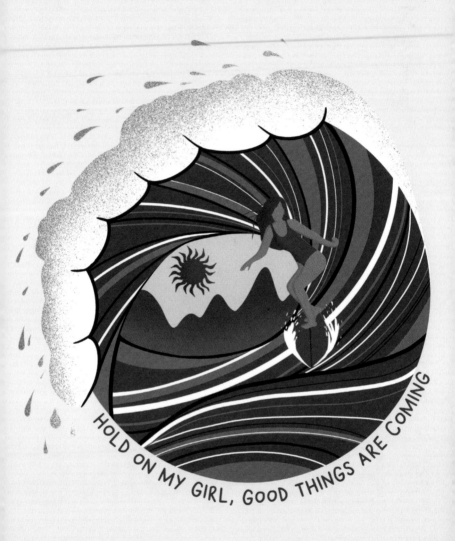

HOLD ON MY GIRL, GOOD THINGS ARE COMING